The #AskDrA Book

Vol 3

Dr. Guillermo Alvarez

The #AskDrA Book

Vol 3

Easy & Practical Answers
To Enjoying Life
As A New "Sleever".

*Based On Episodes 53-78 Of The #AskDrA Show.

The #AskDrA Book - Vol 3

Dedicated

To my son, Guillermo.

Contents

Foreword

Years ago, we didn't have the luxury of being able to view YouTube videos, #AskDrA show and testimonials to gather information be it our patients of other doctor's patients who weren't given information in order to fully understand the magnitude of this surgery and what you need to do to be successful. Even with being a nurse, I have learned so much from this man and am so proud to be a member of the "A" team. It has truly been the best humbling experience and just my dream position. It has been my pleasure to have assisted so many patients that have come our way and welcomed into the Endobariatric family, the experience that you will have when you walk through those doors is one that is hard to explain until you are doing it... and one that you will not regret.

> **Susan George, LVN Patient Coordinator since 2005 and a sleeve patient of Dr. A herself**

Dr. Alvarez and the entire Endobariatric Team is always hard at work to make the ease of The Endobariatric Experience a breeze for not only the patient but the companions as well. This has never gone unrecognized as Susan and myself are constantly reminded what a wonderful experience this has been.

I am from Jonesboro, Arkansas where the name Dr. Alvarez rings a bell because so many in NEA (NorthEast Arkansas) have been sleeved by the "famous" Dr. A! He is known as a hero to so many including myself. He saved me from drowning in my own 400+ pound miserable life. I smiled on the outside but was literally dying on the inside. After my primary care physician along with many others kept cheering me on, I decided to take The Endobariatric Experience myself, all the way to Piedras Negras, Mexico. I am more than ecstatic I had VSG surgery with Dr. Alvarez and The Endobariatric Team. It was truly the experience that everyone said - you really do become family. I am currently down 165 lbs and still pushing to get to my final goals. I am 2 years post op, and feel 10 years younger! I am sure I look it too, lol!

Dr. A's books helped me so much through the first year of my journey. I still find myself pulling the books out from time to time, freshening up on my knowledge as I do help so many others now as Dr. A's patient assistant. I highly recommend all of them from the patient stand point, as well as the person behind the computer assisting patients daily.

Dr. Alvarez explains things about the entire journey in regular people's terms not all that fancy medical talk. It is easy to read, understand and learn!

The first edition published in June of 2016, was such a huge hit for VSG patients just like us. We all had a beginning to our journey and understand that you may have questions unanswered, that you just cannot seem to get your doctor's office to give a solid answer. Dr. Alvarez recognized the need for education with patients both pre-and post-op, that he continued to do The #AskDrA Show for that benefit. He has made what the "real world" makes out to be such a huge deal to an easy practical lifestyle not only for the patient but the family too. These books have so much knowledge about the sleeved life, if you read all 3 then you should have a huge head start on your journey!

Susan, myself and The Endobariatric Team always represent the many disciplines and values that Dr. Alvarez and Endobariatric serves. It is my hope as Dr. Alvarez's patient assistant and coordinator that this book, along with volume 1 & 2, will provide an effective learning experience for you during your own personal VSG journey.

Xoxo,
Brandi Carter, Patient Assistant

Introduction

By: Dr. Guillermo Alvarez

You asked, and we delivered. The #AskDrA Book Volume 3 book is here!

It's thanks to our incredible group of passionate, engaged patients that this book, as well as the ones that proceeded it, were written. Every week, patients from all over the world send us questions that are crucial to their gastric sleeve weight loss journey. And if they have these questions, lots of other people probably do, too. That's why we continue to create these resources.

I'm a true believer that knowledge is power, and this Q&A format is an easy-to-digest way to access important information. This volume delivers the concise info many of you want—the "quick and dirty" answer that allows you get on with your day fast. But we've also provided links at the beginning of each chapter if you'd like more complete information on a topic.

I hope this book proves valuable to you, whether you're pre-op or have been sleeved for years. The more you know about maximizing your gastric sleeve surgery, the better your outcome will be. And that's our goal here at Endobariatric: healthy, happy patients.

If you'd like to join the discussion, simply add the hashtag #AskDrA on social media, and I'll be there to help. Your question might even appear in a future AskDrA book.

See you online!

Dr. Alvarez

Chapter 53

(You'll find Chapters 1 – 52 in the Ask Dr. A Books 1 and 2)

Desire For Desserts, Dumping With Milk & Sodium Consumption

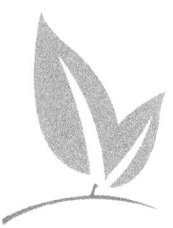

"Having a sleeve is a re-learning process.
It takes time!"

To watch the #AskDrA Show episode that this
chapter is based on, follow along at:
www.bit.ly/AskDrA53

Is it true that our desire for dessert or something sweet after dinner subside after surgery?

That's a very good question. And, the reason I decided to put this one in the book first, is because you need to understand there are two different things here. The first one is the hunger hormone, (or the ghrelin) that is removed in about 80% of stomachs during surgery. With that hunger hormone removed patients soon discover the benefit of not being hungry. Unfortunately, it's very different than the desire you experience for desserts and other foods after surgery.

Yes, desire is the second thing. Because that desire comes from within. It's a learned process. It's something that even though you had surgery, if I tell you, "You know what pizza tastes like," you're going to say, "Yeah." Why? Because you learned what it tastes like. If I tell you, "You know what a cheesesteak tastes like," you're going to say, "Yeah." Because you learned what a cheesesteak tastes like.

Being hungry comes from the body telling you it needs calories, it needs food. The desire comes from your mind. If you don't put that extra effort in, you will have to make it work and get the best out of it, you need to re-learn. Yes, it's a learning process.

I tell patients having a sleeve it's a re-learning process. It takes time, but patients do absolutely amazing and, with the hunger gone, it helps tremendously.

Is it normal to have dumping with milk?

Specifically, on phase two, patients may have a little bit of diarrhea. Patients may experience a little bit of dumping syndrome. We've talked about the dumping syndrome before (in Vol 1 & Vol 2). It's not that common with the sleeve. It is more common with gastric bypass though.

Some patients may experience diarrhea because the osmolarity of the milk, is very thick. It's very rich. It goes down into the sleeve. Before surgery, you had a big pouch of stomach. Your stomach would hold the milk, or the shake, or whatever substance containing lactose. That would stay inside your stomach for a few minutes to an hour. It would slowly drip it into the small intestine. Your body would tolerate it quite easily.

Now, right after surgery, you might start to do shakes. This shake with milk goes directly into the first portion of the intestine and produces osmotic diarrhea, a rapid motility of the intestine and a very similar situation like with dumping syndrome.

What you need to do is try to avoid this situation the first few weeks after surgery. Try other alternatives. If you want to do protein, you can mix it with water.

Try lactose-free products. Work around it and you'll be just fine. Remember, this is just temporary. As the swollen tissue starts to come down, the capacity of your sleeve starts to hold food or liquids a little bit better and longer. Patients are freaking out thinking they're going to have this problem or issue forever. This is just because it's so recent there's not enough space in the sleeve. It goes directly to your intestine and will make you run to the restroom.

How much sodium should we be consuming per day?

The reason I decided to share this question is because I want you to be aware of your sodium consumption. Just to give you a little bit of information, if you consume a teaspoon of salt a day, you're going to be above the daily recommended allowance of sodium. A teaspoon of salt equals about 2,325 milligrams. The daily recommended allowance is 2,300.

It's very important not to add salt to your food. If you cooked with a little bit of salt, keep it that way. If it tastes kind of good, don't add more salt. I see some patients that without even tasting the food, they're grabbing for the salt. Don't do that. Taste your food first.

If you go to a restaurant, they've already added some salt to your food. If your spouse or a friend cooked your meal, it already has some sodium. Try to avoid adding more salt.

Let's talk about processed and canned foods. They contain a lot of sodium because they need to be preserved for longer periods of time. The sodium is very high on these foods, so try to avoid processed foods, canned foods, and of course, using the kitchen table salt.

Chapter 54

Feeling Tired, Diets & Medications We Supply

"Remember this is all temporary, it will get better as your body adapts."

To watch the #AskDrA Show episode that this chapter is based on, follow along at: www.bit.ly/AskDrA54

I'm having trouble doing my job, and can barely keep my eyes open. Any advice?

Here's the most important thing, your mindset. Your body is adapting to the lower calories per day. By the time your surgery comes, and afterwards, you're going to be consuming very small amounts of calories per day. But, if you don't do this diet correctly, you will feel tired. You may feel weak, you may feel lightheaded, you may feel dizzy, because you didn't adapt in the period of time that you should have.

What can you do? Well, check with your doctor. If I'm your doctor, you contact me. You contact me or my coordinator Susan, and we'll be right there. Otherwise, contact your doctor. We need to review what medications you might taking or possibly need. Diabetes, diabetes medication, high blood pressure medicine and a vast majority of medications can cause you to feel weak and tired during the day time.

Make sure you're resting correctly, getting enough sleep. Getting enough carbs and enough calories. Get My Fitness Pal. Download it to your phone, log in. I do it every day.

Log in your calories, your food intake. Log in the amount of food you're in-taking, the water intake. That will help you, and check your medications with your doctor. That will help you to avoid those sensations of being tired, and it will get better. Remember this is all temporary, it will get better as your body adapts.

Why is it important to not only do low carb diet, low calories, but also making sure it is low fat?

Let's get things straight. It's very different to talk about a low carb diet, a low fat diet and a low calorie diet. You're talking about three different concepts. If you're doing low carb, that means you got three things you can use. Either protein, carbs, or fat. If I'm lowering your carb intake, I can't lower your fat intake. You need to do either protein or fat. If you're looking at the low fat diet, of course it's going to be carbs and protein that you're going to be eating. If you're looking now at calories, it's going to be a balanced diet, and you're lowering the amount of calories you're consuming per day.

Again, that's the importance of My Fitness Pal. It will track your calories. I'm not a spokesperson for My Fitness Pal, I'm just trying to help you. I just have the free version. But the pro version can show you the amount of protein you're eating per day, calories by fat, and calories by carbs. It's very useful.

If you're doing low carb, don't focus on the fat. If you're doing a low fat diet, then focus on lowering that fat intake. They're totally different diets. Why do I recommend a low carb, high protein diet? Because it's easy to do. Because it's very accommodating to the American culture tradition of the way we eat. That's why. It works really good.

"But, Dr. Alvarez, but you're a vegan, why would you promote this diet?" Because it's easy to do, and most patients can adapt quite simple.

And, if you want to take it a step further, and try being a vegetarian, a pesco-vegetarian, I mean even go up to being a vegan, you can try it out. It works great because you're getting the most calories from plant based foods. But the vegan diet is much healthier than the low carb diet. Vegan diet is much healthier than the low carb diet. But the low carb diet works really good, because you've got the sleeve restricting the amount of calories you're intaking, and yourself, you're making wise decisions and lowering the amount of calories by carbs. That way you're going to be melting the fat off. Please, just to get things straight, you got those three diets. Don't mix the concepts up.

Do you supply all the prescriptions we need after surgery?

If you decide to come to us for surgery, we take care of you from the get go. All you have to do is get yourselves to San Antonio. We take care of transportation, hotel, logistics, hospital bills, doctor fees, even the medications you go home with. We give you the prescription, and we fill it out for you.

You don't have to worry about anything. We'll take you back to San Antonio, leave you there for an extra night in a nice hotel, and then you can take your flight back home. Everything's included in the package. Yeah, we supply every single medication that is prescribed, and that you need going back home.

Chapter 55

Aspirin, Mood Swings, Appetite Suppressants

"Remember that you did this procedure to change your lifestyle. Make wise decisions. Don't fill up your sleeve with junk food."

To watch the #AskDrA Show episode that this chapter is based on, follow along at: www.bit.ly/AskDrA55

I haven't taken Aspirin since before surgery. Should I go back on it at some point?

Aspirin belongs to a category called non steroid anti-inflammatories. NSAIDS. We talked about this before. These medications are very rough on a regular stomach. They can make the stomach bleed. They can create ulcers. Now let's talk about an operated stomach (gastric bypass, gastric sleeve). Even rougher. We need to avoid these medications. Talk to your surgeon about taking these medications.

Now let's say your doctor, your cardiologist insists that you take aspirin. You can, but no sooner than 21 days after surgery, but I wouldn't take the 500 mg per day. Nor the 325 per day. I would take the 81 milligram per day and make sure you're taking an acid blocker morning and evening, or something to protect your stomach while you're taking this medication.

I'm having terrible mood swings. Is this normal?

Mood swings are normal. But sometimes it has to do with the amount of calories you're intaking. Make sure you're intaking enough per day and that you're logging in your calories, as we talked about previously. At least 600 to 800 calories per day, plus enough carbs. Also check your medications. Some medications can cause mood swings. Again just temporary. It's your body going through a lot of adjustments. It'll pass.

Can I take an appetite suppressant?

This is a very common question for sleevers. Now you're a few months out from surgery and you really want to crush it. You think about taking appetite suppressants because you're getting those cravings for junk food. Remember that you did this procedure to change your lifestyle. Make wise decisions. Don't fill up your sleeve with junk food. You got a craving? Fill it up with a fruit. Banana, pear, grape. No junk food.

If you want to take appetite suppressants, can you? The answer is yes. It won't cause any problems to your sleeve. I wouldn't recommend it though. Just try to make wiser decisions. Help your sleeve, and you'll get the most out of it.

Chapter 56

How To Lose 100 Pounds, Burping & Anti-Inflammatories

"You do need to work with it and make wise decisions."

To watch the #AskDrA Show episode that this chapter is based on, follow along at: www.bit.ly/AskDrA56

What is the fastest way to lose 100 pounds?

Get gastric sleeve surgery! Is it that simple? Of course not. Remember that the sleeve is a tool, but it's a very powerful tool that will help you get to that goal. Set small goals. Set achievable goals. Little by little, lose the first 20 pounds, then the next 20 or 30 pounds, then move up to 70 pounds. By the time you know it, you've completed the task of losing 100 pounds.

You do need to work with it and make wise decisions. It's important for you to understand that the sleeve is not magical. But once you understand how to use that tool you lose 100 pounds, 150 pounds, 200 pounds or more.

Why does the sleeve cause you to belch as soon as you eat or drink?

The burping is caused because the sleeve is swollen and a little bit of air gets trapped along the pathway of the sleeve. If you move, or you drink a little bit of fluid or you eat a little bit of food, that passage frees up, and that air flows up, and you burp. If you take your antacid, that will help open up the space, and then there's that free flow of air, or that column of air that will actually eliminate that burping sensation.

What about occasional use of Meloxicam?

Meloxicam is one of the most common anti- inflammatories used, especially for muscular aches, knee pain, lower back pain, et cetera. You can take it just for a short period of time, same as ibuprofen.

There are other options. Instead of taking Meloxicam, you can take Celebrex, which is easier on your stomach, on your sleeve. You can also check with your surgeon for other possibilities or other medications that you can use instead of the anti-inflammatories.

Chapter 57

Food Cravings, Plastic Surgery & The Paleo Diet

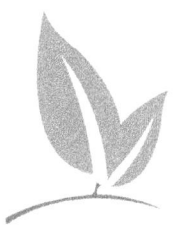

"If there's something in that ingredient list that you can't pronounce or have no idea what it is, then it does not go into your diet."

To watch the #AskDrA Show episode that this chapter is based on, follow along at: www.bit.ly/AskDrA57

Is it possible to have food cravings after surgery?

Yes of course. It has nothing to do with the ghrelin hormone that goes away after you have gastric sleeve surgery. We talked about this. It's a learned experience.

But, what science has proven is that your head hunger and your cravings are reduced about 80% after surgery. And this reduction will help you in losing the weight and help you focus on staying on track with your weight loss goals.

When do you think its the best time to have the plastic surgery?

When to have plastic surgery. Number one, talk to your plastic surgeon. But not until, and this is number two, wait until you've plateaued. Once you're at a good stable weight, you're at your goal for a couple of months. No sooner than 12 months or 18 months, depending on your excess weight and when you've hit goal.

But, let's say you're a low BMI patient, 35 or a little under, and you've lost the weight really quick, you might be able to see the plastic surgeon in seven to ten months. You don't have to wait 18 months to have plastic surgery.

Talk to your plastic surgeon, he will evaluate you. He can actually coordinate with your bariatric surgeon and then come to a conclusion which is best for you. Although in normal conditions no sooner than 12 to 18 months.

What's your opinion on following the paleo diet?

Let's talk a little bit about the paleo diet. Paleo diet is very similar to the low carb diet. It actually mimics the diet that prehistoric civilization would eat. Some call it the cave man diet. You eat meat, you can eat fish, you can eat fruits and vegetables. Nothing processed.

Nowadays, the food industry has a whole array of processed stuff available for easy picking in your super market. But you have to look at the labeling and look at the ingredients. If there's something in that ingredient list that you can't pronounce or have no idea what it is, then it does not go into the paleo diet, it's quite simple.

What do I think? Sounds okay, right? I'm not saying it's the healthiest thing you can eat because you're eating a whole bunch of animal products which I don't care for in my diet. But, let me tell you this, if it works for you and you see results, then it's fine. But for me, personal opinion, eating too much of those animal products is not a good way to go because it will give you a quite a bit of side effects down the road, triglycerides, cholesterol, insulin resistance, and so forth. But of course, your sleeve will limit the amount of food intake.

You can always touch base with your nutritionist in conjunction with your bariatric surgeon and they can work together of what's a good diet plan for you.

Chapter 58

Aches And Pains, Eating And Drinking & Oatmeal

"Time will give you the pace. Be patient."

To watch the #AskDrA Show episode that this
chapter is based on, follow along at:
www.bit.ly/AskDrA58

Is there any other type of medication you can take for a headache besides Tylenol?

Tylenol is a very important ally when aches and pains arise after your sleeve because Tylenol is very mild and does not interfere with your stomach's lining. So any other medication that's called an anti- inflammatory (for example: nonsteroidal anti- inflammatory, and we talked about NSAIDs before) does affect the lining of the stomach and may be harmful if used several times a day or for a long period of time, which is called chronic use.

But let's say it's for a regular headache and that Tylenol just doesn't do the work. So what you can do is, take some Advil, or some Ibuprofen which would be the next option. Don't take Aspirin, please, Aspirin is really rough on the stomach. Don't take Naproxen, it too is really rough on the stomach.

For menstrual cramps, ladies can use it once a month, that's fine. Twice, two days continuously, that's fine. But for longer periods of time, it may harm your sleeve so you need to be very careful. That's why your number one option, is Tylenol.

Can I never eat and drink together again?

Will you be able to eat and drink at the same time? The answer is yes. Normally the first few months, it's practically impossible because there isn't enough room in that new sleeve. It's a very narrow tube and either food goes in there or some liquids. When you eat and drink at same time they will compete for that space and that liquid will go down and switch places with that food, it's a very uncomfortable sensation. You may feel some pressure in your chest and some other sensations that you may not like. That's about it. There is no other risk.

Your sleeve will not blow up, your sleeve will not be harmed at all. It's just, what we're trying to do is avoid these uncomfortable sensations. Once the swollen tissue comes down, the inflammation comes down and following, let's say, six months or even longer, maybe a year, you'll be able to drink and eat together. Time will give you the pace. Be patient.

Can we ever eat oatmeal again?

During your post-op phase, you may notice that there are some types of food that may not agree with you. What we experienced in the last 11 years doing the sleeve is that some people may have a hard time with rice. Maybe some people have a hard time with bread, and some people have a hard time with oatmeal. Why is this? Because some types of food do grab more moisture and expand in the stomach. Such is the case of oatmeal. If you leave oatmeal, put some water in it, and just leave it for a few minutes, actually that oatmeal will grab the moisture from the water, pull it in and expand. Same goes for bread, may go also with some rice, et cetera.

So when that happens, you may have an uncomfortable sensation. Will it go away? The answer is yes. You have to give it some time. At a certain point, you will be able to tolerate these types of foods, and all you have to do in the meantime is just identify what types of food go well with you and your sleeve.

Chapter 59

Taking Capsules, Midnight Cravings & Dry Heaving

"Balance the calories throughout the day and those cravings will disappear."

To watch the #AskDrA Show episode that this chapter is based on, follow along at: www.bit.ly/AskDrA59

Can I swallow capsules?

Yes, you can. Remember that capsules are not as big as an issue as the solid pills. Capsules have that enteric coating, and when you swallow the capsules, they hit the stomach, they disintegrate and release the medication. No problem there at all. So regarding pills, yes you can take those too, but, you got to be careful. Pills, and this is our rule, should be no bigger than an M&M candy. We're talking about the plain ones, not the peanut ones, okay, got it? If bigger than a regular M&M, you'll have to cut them in half. Capsules though, shouldn't be a problem. Check with your doctor first and he/she will advise further.

What can I do to curb midnight cravings?

This is actually very easy. All you have to do, is balance your calories throughout the day and you won't have those cravings. But, if you skip a meal, skip a breakfast, skip lunch, or even have a late lunch, then the cravings come in later in the evening. So what you have to do, balance things off. Balance the calories throughout the day and those cravings will disappear. So in the morning have your breakfast, at noon have your lunch, in the evening your dinner. And if you you need some snacking mid-morning, mid-afternoon, that's okay. It'll be easy. Do it, and let me know how it goes.

Is dry heaving damaging to your sleeve immediately after surgery?

The answer is no. I tell patients you could be throwing up 20, 30 times a day, and you still won't damage the sleeve, it won't cause any issues. The sleeve will get swollen, yeah, but it won't make the sleeve rupture or burst or anything like that. So, put your mind at ease. The reason we included this question, well, I got an email from this patient that had a spell of dry heaving. And she was freaking out. She thought she might have damaged the sleeve. The answer is no. Even right after surgery, the day following surgery, or even the day of surgery, it won't be an issue.

In the take-home medication we give to our patients we include anti-nausea pills. A small percentage of patients use them. It's just not something that most patients experience, just small minority. So put your mind at ease.

Chapter 60

Breath Mints, Diet Soft Drinks & Tailbone Pain

"Drop the carbonation. It will be easier to then progress to tea to plain water."

To watch the #AskDrA Show episode that this chapter is based on, follow along at: www.bit.ly/AskDrA60

Can you have breath mints shortly after surgery?

This is a very common question that we get in the hospital, not before surgery. It's normally the day of the surgery, you may have a little dry mouth sensation and patients are eager to have something. And they sometimes say, "can I have a breath mint?" In our practice we don't allow them the first 24 hours after surgery.

Why? Well, we want that stomach dry until the next day. Then we'll start you off with ice chips. The cold and moisture of the ice brings the swollen stomach tissue down.

But the breath mints, we try to avoid them. We do recommend our patients use swabs, and when brushing their teeth they can rinse with some water. It helps with the dry mouth sensation. But remember you're going to be well hydrated with your IV. It's just that sensation, the dry mouth sensation, that you can use other tricks and tips besides what is being mentioned here to help you with that sensation.

Is Coke Zero better than other diet drinks?

The answer is they're all bad and crappy. Try to avoid soft drinks.

Try by lowering your consumption daily if you're drinking a whole bunch of Diet Coke or Diet Zero or diet whatever. They 're just bad for you. Try to avoid carbonated beverages altogether.

Drop the carbonation. It will be easier to then progress to Crystal Light or tea to plain water.

Is the weight loss a contributing factor if I have issues with major tailbone pain?

Alright so this question we can use two ways. I have tailbone pain, will this get better or worse once I have weight loss surgery? Well, terrible pain (if you have it right now) will continue even after surgery. The other question is can I get tailbone pain after weight loss surgery? The answer is yes because that fatty cushion is starting to go away.

Yes, it will get a little uncomfortable if you already have tailbone pain. Normally, it's not something we see on every patient, but if you do have it, will it continue? Yeah.

Chapter 61

Eating And Drinking, Heartburn & Getting Back On Track

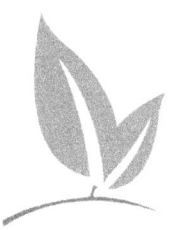

"You need to schedule it. You need to put it on your phone, schedule your agenda and put in your exercise time."

To watch the #AskDrA Show episode that this chapter is based on, follow along at: www.bit.ly/AskDrA61

When do I need to stop drinking fluids before and after meals? During the soft food phase or when I'm eating regular food?

It's when you're starting to eat soft foods. That is important. You'll notice that if you drink fluids with your meals, even though it's soft food, it may produce this uncomfortable sensation.

Soft-food phase, stop the drinking 30 minutes before the meals, your solid meals, and you can resume fluids 30 minutes after. It's soft foods, not the regular foods, all right? Be careful with the eating and drinking at the same time.

How long does heartburn last after surgery?

It's important to mention that not everybody gets heartburn after surgery. It's normally seen with patients that have had heartburn, or GERD, gastroesophageal reflux disease, in the past. This is commonly seen in those patients, not in new patients, or patients who don't have heartburn or don't have that history. Now, let's say, you don't have that history of heartburn and you do get some heartburn, or indigestion, or GERD, how long does it last? Just to mention that the heartburn, or indigestion, or sometimes the "hunger sensations" some people feel right after surgery, some people say, "I'm hungry I thought this surgery was supposed to put the fire out, put the hunger away, because you're cutting off that ghrelin hormone, the hormone that produces hunger, and why am I hungry right after surgery?"

The deal is that the stomach has just been manipulated, it just had been stapled, over sewn, and this produces a lot of inflammation and swollen tissue on the stomach. That swollen tissue, your brain detects that as hunger, so it doesn't mean that you're really hungry, it's just it's so swollen that your brain detects it that you need food or you're hungry. That is why, in every regular practice, you'll be given some antacids or acid blockers, to put that fire out. It is very important. I tell patients that this the most important medication you're going home with. When you return home, it's that acid blocker that you'll twice a day because it helps to put that swollen tissue down, and that sensation goes away.

Just to let you know, that this sensation, or this symptom, is temporary, and it goes away in the following days after surgery. After surgery when you wake up, or a day or two after, and you feel "hungry", remember that the stomach is so swollen because you just had major surgery just a few hours ago. Now, after surgery, let's say seven days out from surgery, you shouldn't have the heartburn or indigestion because, in theory, you're taking the acid blockers. If you're not, get yourself back on track, take your medications, and you'll be just fine.

I have gone off the good path a little and now I'm having trouble getting back on, what advice would you give?

How to get back on track. There's certain things you need to do. If you know that you have fallen off the wagon and you're off track. You know exactly in what aspects you're having an issue with, so you need to attack those problems, you need to address those issues that are getting you off track. It's very important.

Number one, is identify these issues, these problems. Is it because you are eating junk food again? If that's the problem, you'll have to stop buying the junk food. When you go to the supermarket, just don't add it to your shopping cart. If you don't buy it, there's no way you can eat it. It's very important to make wise decisions there.

"I stopped exercising, because I didn't have a good regimen and I fell off the wagon, I need to get back on track". You need to think, what is causing the problem here? Is it lack of time? Is it you being busy or just making up excuses? Because excuses, they're always there. You can always make up some excuse that can move that exercise time later in the day. You need to schedule it. You need to put it on your phone, schedule your agenda and put in your exercise time.

It's like you're meeting your local mayor, your meeting the president of your nation. If that is a time you've scheduled it, there's nothing more important than that time, because it's more important than the President of the United States, it's you. It's time for you. You need to make that time for yourself, so if you don't make it, nobody else is going to be making that time of the day to exercise. You need to create it.

Once you create that time of the day, you need to respect it, and do it. Now, you're starting off slow, that's fine, it doesn't matter, as long as you're keeping a log, and you're inputing the amount of times you've exercised and how you've been increasing this endurance, it's great, you get motivated.

Number two, it also gives you the opportunity to log in your exercise, and that's really cool because you know when you did your exercise, how you've been progressing, or increasing your endurance, or where you stand, so it's quite simple. There's option number three that's really cool, because you can also log in your water, and we've talked about logging in water. If you don't know how much you're doing, you're not keeping track, there's no way, you're lost. You need to keep track of your water intake. That application is really complete, it's very good, and very easy and useful to handle. It's very handy to have on your phone.

Chapter 62

Types of Exercise, Who's Eligible & Pregnancy

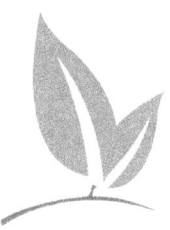

"After sleeve surgery combine a little bit of the cardio with the weight resistance to keep tone and fit."

To watch the #AskDrA Show episode that this chapter is based on, follow along at: www.bit.ly/AskDrA62

What exercises would you recommend to tone up as much as possible before skin removal surgery?

Let's talk about types of exercise to get the best results down the road with your sleeve to avoid the loose skin. I like to recommend to my patients the elliptical machine. It gives you the movement which is cardiovascular, but it also tones your upper body. It works really well. Patients do really good because they're toning, at the same time doing their cardio. But if you really want to get toned up, you can do the elliptical machine with a little bit of weight resistance and that gives the best results. If you talk to a personal trainer, they'll tell you about this. They'll try to combine a little bit of the cardio with the weight resistance. But the weight resistance has to be low weight, very high reps. That's the key. But of course the personal trainers will tell you this.

Would a patient be eligible it they are not very overweight, but have always struggled to keep the weight off?

Do we have to be really big to be a candidate for the sleeve or eligible for the sleeve? Or do you have to be really overweight? Like 300, 400 pounds, 500 pounds or more. The answer is no. You could be 200 pounds. You can be even less than 200 pounds and still be eligible for the sleeve. It all depends on BMI, body mass index. You can Google BMI calculators on line. There's a ton of them that show up.

Normally a BMI of 35 and over are considered candidates. Sometimes BMI between 30 and 35 depending on medical conditions may be eligible for gastric sleeve surgery. It all depends on the BMI, and what your surgeon can dictate. Of course we have an online form that you can fill out. And yes, I go over these forms personally and will let you know if you are eligible or not.

How does pregnancy affect your weight loss if you are still losing weight? How does it compare to having the surgery after pregnancy?

Pregnancy after the sleeve is very safe. You'll be fine. The baby will be fine. Actually it will be better because having a pregnancy while being overweight can put you and the baby at a much higher risks. You need to be aware that once you lose the weight or you're losing the weight, it's much better for you and the baby. Nutrition wise, it doesn't affect the baby. We have a ton of sleeve babies so far. We have them ever year. Last year I had a patient who delivered triplets. She's fine. The babies were fine. All you have to do is focus on the nutrition aspect. Make sure you're taking your maternal vitamins and you're following up with your OB/GYN.

But of course, every once in a while, include your bariatric surgeon in the game here. It's important. The vast majority of the patients once they deliver the baby, that baby fat goes away really quick. Fast, easy and effective. You don't stick to those extra pounds. In a short sentence, it's safe for you, safe for the baby. It's even safer than when you were overweight.

Chapter 63

Quinoa, Lump Under An Incision & Shakes Causing Nausea

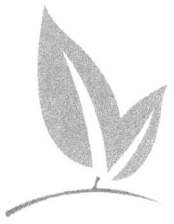

"If you're looking for something healthy, good for you, a super food, quinoa is a deal."

To watch the #AskDrA Show episode that this chapter is based on, follow along at: www.bit.ly/AskDrA63

Let's talk about quinoa.
Take it or leave it?

Take it, take it. Unless, you are looking into counting carbs, quinoa does have carbs. You need to look out for that. If you're doing a low carb diet, look into some other choices instead of the quinoa, but if you're looking for something healthy, good for you, a super food, quinoa is a deal. It's a source of good protein, fiber, and you should take it.

Is it normal to have a hard lump under the incision site?

So you have a lump under one of the incisions, normally it would be the extraction point. With our patients, left side, biggest incision, that's where the portion of the stomach comes out. We do a lot more manipulation right there and a lump may form right under that incision. If you touch every single incision, you'll feel little lumps because that's part of the healing process. You'll have inflammation. Look at it as a human cement, all right? Human cement, it's forming, it's hard. Over time that hardening starts to become soft and it goes away. The first four to six weeks people, totally normal, don't freak out. It's not a hernia. It's not an alien coming out of your body. It's totally normal and it'll become soft as the rest of your abdominal wall heals. Patience, right there.

Is it normal that my protein drinks are making me nauseated?

If your protein shakes cause nausea, what do you have to do? The simple solution...switch brands. Or find some other alternative instead of sticking to those protein shakes. I understand, some protein shakes could taste kind of nasty. You need to try to work around it, try a different brand. Maybe try it a different form. If you're doing it with milk, maybe try lactose free, maybe try a skim, maybe try with water. You need to look out for a different brand that works for you. Don't think that every, every protein shake will cause some nausea and you need to look for an alternative. It's not a rule that a protein shake equals nausea. No, there's some that I really enjoy.

Chapter 64

Stopping Weight Loss At Goal, Stalls & What To Do Before Surgery

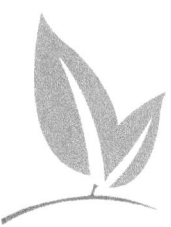

"The more weight you lose at the beginning of your weight lose journey, the less weight you need to lose down the road."

To watch the #AskDrA Show episode that this chapter is based on, follow along at: www.bit.ly/AskDrA64

Once you reach your weight loss goals, how do you stop losing weight?

All right, so it's not a very frequent question that you get. Like, "What am I going to do once I reach goal?" It's normally a pre-op patient, a pre-op question from a patient that's looking into the sleeve and is thinking, "Well, once I reached goal, what do I supposed to do, or how does my body know that I've reached goal and not to lose too much weight?" Doesn't work like that.

Remember, the sleeve will advance really quick the first few to 12 months. The more weight you lose at the beginning of your weight lose journey, the less weight you need to lose down the road. Your body burns less calories when you don't have to move that much mass around. So your body weighs less, and you burn less calories. So you'll have really fast weight loss right away, because the sleeve will kick- start your metabolism.

Remember that the sleeve is a portion of stomach. The surgeon doesn't go, "Well, I'll just cut here, and here, and here, and here, and that should work. That should make the magic happen." No, it's a calibrated sleeve. It's a calibration that we use during surgery, to leave that stomach a certain size.

So even though the sleeve is a tool. You need to work with it. The sleeve will not be calibrated like a dial. It doesn't happen that way. Watch what you eat, exercise daily and your body will adjust to where it needs to be.

How long is too long of a stall?

Weight stalls are normal, so you need to understand they are needed for the body to adjust to the new you, to the new size, to your new weight, to your new amount of fluid in your body, to the amount your body metabolizes everything. Even to the amount of blood in your bloodstream. Everything changes depending on your weight. So your body puts on that emergency brake on, hits a stall. It's intended, and needed. And then your body adjusts, and that's when patients notice they start losing sizes.

And so, how long is too long for a stall? It depends, everyone is different. There is no exact number. I can't tell you, "one week" or "four weeks" or, "five weeks".

Any recommendations on things I should be doing to prepare for surgery?

Follow your surgeon's guidelines. In our practice, we have everything for you. We have a shopping list for things to have at home once you get back from surgery. You've got things to do before surgery. You've got a list on what to bring for surgery. Everything is already set up for my patients. Probably the most important thing, probably the best advice I can give you, is to follow the pre-op diet to the tee.

Chapter 65

Ghrelin, Omega 3 & Osteoarthritis

"With the gastric sleeve you will be a fat-burning machine."

To watch the #AskDrA Show episode that this chapter is based on, follow along at: www.bit.ly/AskDrA65

After some time, does the ghrelin that was removed during surgery regenerate?

If you don't know what the ghrelin hormone is, that is a hormone that produces hunger. That hormone is found in your stomach and small intestine. During gastric sleeve surgery we remove 75-80% of your stomach, which cuts down on the ghrelin being produced.

So it's not removed completely. Thing is, right after surgery you do notice that the ghrelin hormone is decreased greatly. That means you're not hungry. Cravings also start to go away. But down the road, as the years go by, you may say, "Well, now I notice that I eat more." Which is different than being hungry, if you're eating more.

The other thing is, you may think you're hungry but it could be that your stomach is swollen. The common thing I see, whether a patient with a sleeve or without a sleeve, is that feeling of being hungry is caused by caffeine, skipping meals, stress, alcohol, smoking, medications you're taking...oh, it's a long list and I could go on and on.

The swollen tissue, your brain detects it as hunger, and guess what? You start eating more, and you're saying, "Well, now I'm hungrier than I used to be before surgery."

It's not the ghrelin regenerating, in most cases your stomach is just swollen.

Is it okay to take Omega-3 to burn fat faster?

Well, the thing is, there are some studies that have shown that taking Omega-3 may help burn fat faster. The thing is, you really don't need it. With the gastric sleeve you will be a fat-burning machine.

So instead of taking Omega-3, do me a favor. Get on the elliptical machine for ten, 15 minutes, or get on the treadmill for 20, 30 minutes, and build it up from there. The way you'll feel, the boost to metabolism, burning fat much higher rate than taking Omega-3.

Can you discuss how surgery helps those with osteoarthritis, especially in the knees?

It's actually very simple. If you have 35, 50, 100, 150 pounds or more to lose, that weight directly effects your knees, your hips and your joints. Every step you take that extra weight is causing harm to your body.

So of course losing this weight will help tremendously. Your body will thank you for it. Your knees will thank you for it. Not just your knees though, your hips, your ankles, everything. I mean, everything gets so much better. We get a lot of referrals from the orthopedic surgeons, people who need knee replacements, hip replacements. And those patients actually can postpone those procedures, even cancel them, just by having weight loss surgery, and losing the weight. I mean, their quality of life gets so much better.

Chapter 66

What Vegetables To Eat, Stalls After A Month & Calories

"Don't freak out. Remember, this is a long journey of 12, 18 months. You need patience here."

To watch the #AskDrA Show episode that this chapter is based on, follow along at:
www.bit.ly/AskDrA66

What are some of the best veggies with the best nutritional value for us with sleeves?

If you're interested in eating more vegetables, or in becoming more like a vegetarian, or adapting to the vegan lifestyle, then yes, there are some vegetables that will give you more nutrients. As you know, I've been vegan for almost over a year and a half or so. Back to the question, the cruciferous group of vegetables will give you the most amount of nutrients, most amount of antioxidants as well. You're talking about cabbage, cauliflower, broccoli, and most importantly, kale.

Is it "normal," knowing that every journey is different, to have my first stall one month after surgery?

Stalls are expected. If you're freaking out, if you had a stall after a month, this is totally normal. Sometimes it comes sooner than a month, because it all depends at what point you started to lose weight before surgery, your pre-op diet, and your starting weight, your age, your activity level. It all comes into play here. Remember, your body's going under a lot of transformation. It needs these stalls for your body to shrink down, to lose the sizes, to adapt to your body functions, and then continue. Don't freak out. Remember, this is a long journey of 12, 18 months. You need patience here.

How many calories and carbs are we supposed to be eating starting soft food?

Let me give you a little bit of the rounded numbers here. Right after post-op, between month one and six, you'll probably be doing between 600 to 800 calories a day. After six months, you'll probably pick it up between 800 to 1000 calories per day, it stays that way for maybe a year, year and a half, then it could go up to 1,200 calories or so. It all depends if you're a man or a woman. Men have larger stomachs. It all depends on your surgeon and their surgical technique. It also has a lot to do with the the bougie calibration tube your surgeon used. All these issues come into play on the amount of calories that you will be consuming afterwards.

Chapter 67

Hair Loss, How Much To Eat & Regain Weight After Surgery

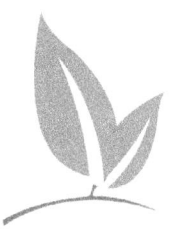

"You need to focus on your protein, take your supplements and just keep focused and everything will be normal."

To watch the #AskDrA Show episode that this chapter is based on, follow along at: www.bit.ly/AskDrA67

How much hair loss is normal?

The average person loses between sixty and a hundred hairs per day. Unfortunately, I lose a little bit more than that and it's starting to show. Weight- loss surgery does not equal hair loss. Having weight-loss surgery or sleeve surgery does not mean you will go bald. But people who have drastic and rapid weight loss will experience a little bit of hair thinning. This is temporary.

You need to focus on your protein, take your supplements and just keep focused and everything will be normal. Every single hair will regrow back, and as I like to say, "I've never seen a bald bariatric patient yet". Your hair will regrow so put your mind at ease. It does not regrow on me, unfortunately, but it will regrow back on you. So don't worry if it starts to shed, push your protein, push your supplements, keep focused, remember this is temporary and as soon as your weight starts to stabilize, it'll regrow again.

What is the approximate volume of food that should be eaten in one meal?

This will vary from surgeon to surgeon, surgical technique to surgical technique, it will also vary from gender. Males get to eat a little bit more than women because males have a slightly larger stomach than females. It also has to do with the calibration tube that is used during surgeries. So, the wider the calibration tube used for surgery, the more you'll be able to eat per meal.

There is no precise measurement because everybody is different. But once you feel full, once you feel that sensation that you're getting full, stop! Get away from the table. Don't push it. Take care of your sleeve, don't over distend your sleeve. Don't overeat.

After such major weight loss, how much do people regain?

How do people regain the weight if they lost so much weight to begin with? It's quite simple. They fall off the wagon, they lose focus.

Remember that if you lost so much weight before you've got to work with your sleeve to get you back there. It's your turn to keep it at that point, you don't want to regain that weight back. But say you lost focus and fell off the wagon and whatever just crosses your plate you just eat. You say to yourself, "I've got a sleeve, I had weight-loss surgery, it's okay for me to eat it, it's no problem, I don't need to watch my calories, I don't need to watch my carbs." It doesn't work that way.

You have to be conscious of what you're eating, how much you're eating. You have to exercise. You need to bust your butt off to burn a hundred or two hundred calories. If you don't track of what you're eating and how you're exercising the weight will come back.

Chapter 68

Ketogenic Diet, Preventing Strictures & Ounces Your Sleeve Holds

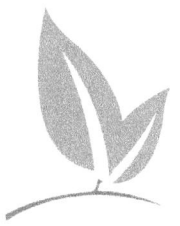

"Once you hit goal, the idea is to lower your fat intake, especially saturated fats."

To watch the #AskDrA Show episode that this chapter is based on, follow along at:
www.bit.ly/AskDrA68

What are your thoughts on a ketogenic diet?

What's my opinion on it? It's a really good diet. It's probably the diet that gives you the fastest results in the shortest amount of time. It's a diet that works on lowering your carb intake, in other words, your sugars. The only thing is...it's not that healthy for you. You're eating a lot of fats and a lot of protein derived from animal products. But it does work really well. I push my patients toward a low carb diet or very similar to the ketogenic diet. Why? Well, because it's very easy for a sleeve patient to follow this diet.

But, once you hit goal, the idea is to lower your fat intake, especially saturated fats. That's when I recommend changing to a plant based diet.

What is a stricture, and are they preventable?

In simple terms a stricture is actually a narrowing. That's it. Imagine an hour glass, you have the top, the middle and the bottom. The middle is that narrow part. You see that stricture coming in, and then it comes out. That narrowing is what we call a stricture in your sleeve.

Is there a way to prevent them? Really, they're not that common. Don't freak out. If you're looking into a gastric sleeve, you're thinking going to get a stricture. No. They're normally associated with high productions of acid or a bad surgical technique or other factors.

You will not be able to prevent that stricture if it was a really bad surgical technique. Normally strictures can be treated endoscopically, which means an endoscopy through the mouth with a little sedation, and a balloon is passed to that part of the stricture, through that narrowing, and we pump air in that balloon, and it actually inflates that stricture. Normally a few sessions, two, three, four sessions, takes care of the problem, and it gets resolved. But that's extreme, again they're not very common.

How many ounces does our stomach hold once we have the sleeve?

It actually varies. But, the average is 4-6 ounces. There are a lot of variables that come into play. The other thing is, men have longer stomachs, and the capacity is slightly larger.

The other thing during the surgical technique, during your surgery, we normally use a calibration tube, and depending on what size that calibration tube was used, that will determine the capacity of your sleeve.

Does your surgeon have enough experience on this procedure and this matter? Does he know exactly what he or she is doing? How many has he or she done and the outcomes they have? Because if they're doing a really wide sleeve, well the capacity will be more, and of course, the success rate will be lower.

Chapter 69

Fruit After Surgery, Setting A Weight Goal & Binge Eating

"The sleeve is a tool, but if used wisely, it will give you enormous potential."

To watch the #AskDrA Show episode that this chapter is based on, follow along at: www.bit.ly/AskDrA69

Is it normal to have difficulties eating fruits?

The answer is no, but it depends at what stage. That is the question here. If you recently jumped from full liquids to soft food, or soft food to regular food, at that phase, you may have some difficulty with certain fruits.

Let's say three months, six months, eight months down the road, if you have difficulties let your doctor know. Maybe there's something wrong. Maybe there isn't. Maybe just need the antacid to calm the swelling and create a little bit more space or room in there.

Patients normally don't have trouble eating fruits after surgery, but it depends at what phase.

How do you know when you have reached goal, if you were never given a goal?

How to set a goal weight? Go by your BMI (Body Mass Index). It's the easiest way to do this. Google BMI calculator. If you don't know which one to choose, we have one on our website at endobariatric.com.

You can type in your height and your current weight, and it will give a BMI score. Aim for a BMI of 25. That would your goal weight. If you get to BMI 25, you would be a normal weight range, all right? Remember that a normal BMI should be between 19 and 25. Between 25 to 29.9 you're overweight. Over 30, you're obese. Over 35, severe obesity. Over 40, morbid obesity. Over 50, super obesity. Over 60, super, super obesity.

Your goal is to be under 25.

Do people still struggle with the desire to overeat after surgery?

Now after surgery, let's say you do have this eating disorder. You're getting treated by it. Let's say a patient with a binge eating disorder has a sleeve. What would happen? Patients are less hungry.

Let's say, for sake of argument, they decide to have a binge eating attack. They want to sit down and just eat to a point that creates an uncomfortable sensation. Well, the thing is, that same sensation that they would feel by eating, let's say a bag of potato chips, and dip. Well, now it's going to be reduced in portion to about a third. The sleeve will be continue helping these people out. It's going to stop them. It's got that emergency brake. Without going overboard to eating the whole amount that they used to eat when they didn't have the sleeve.

Remember, binge eating is an eating disorder that needs treatment. The sleeve works because it's got that brake always on and that won't let you go overboard. If you still eat a lot with the sleeve, you will create or reproduce this uncomfortable sensation that was reproduced, of course, even before surgery.

Remember, I've said it again. The sleeve is a tool, but if used wisely, it will give you enormous potential.

Chapter 70

Protein Shakes, Sleeving Young Adults & Vegetable Protein

"Once you lose the weight, you'll have a much better quality of life, which is the goal here."

To watch the #AskDrA Show episode that this chapter is based on, follow along at: www.bit.ly/AskDrA70

What can I do if my protein shake says not to use for weight reduction?

Now first of all, about protein shakes, I recommend them the first few phases after your surgery. After you start eating, you should drop the protein shakes.

If the protein shake is labeled not for weight reduction, don't worry about it. We're using the shake for nutrition only. Supplemental nutrition. That's it.

What is your overall view of the results and success of the gastric sleeve on a young adult?

Young adults have better metabolism. And will have much better results than older adults.

Don't worry about if I'm getting the sleeve at an older age. You're getting the surgery to have a better quality of life, have better life, to live longer. Whether you can get your sleeve done as a teenager, a young adult or an older adult, you'll do fantastic.

Once you lose the weight, you'll have a much better quality of life, which is the goal here.

Am I going to have any problems getting my protein in after surgery because I don't eat meat?

Should you worry how you're going to get the protein intake if you don't eat meat? No, there are several other sources, right after surgery. We just talked about the protein shakes that you're going to be using as a nutritional supplement. Further down the road, you can also do fish, chicken, turkey, or if you're even thinking of becoming a vegan or you're a vegan, you can get your protein out of your vegetables. It's a vegetable protein source that will get you the amount of protein needed for your body to just work perfectly fine.

Don't worry. There are several options for you. If you have any questions, contact your surgeon, contact me, and we can always help you out.

Chapter 71

Counting Carbs, Our Practice & Hiatal Hernia

"If you are following a low carb diet you should stay away from natural sweeteners or natural sugars."

To watch the #AskDrA Show episode that this chapter is based on, follow along at: www.bit.ly/AskDrA71

When counting carbs, do you include natural sugars from fruits and vegetables?

If you're counting carbs, should you look out for natural sugars found in vegetables, found in fruits? The answer is yes. If you are following a low carb diet you should stay away from natural sweeteners or natural sugar, in this case fructose found in fruits. Yes, you need to do take them into account, because they do contain quite a bit of carbs. If you're looking at lowering your carb intake you need to count the amount of grams of carbs found in vegetables and in fruits.

Does your clinic only perform gastric sleeve and why not bypass?

In our practice, we have focused only and solely on the gastric sleeve procedure for the last 4-5 years. Why not the gastric bypass? Well, it's a more invasive procedure. It's a procedure that takes longer to perform. It's a procedure that comes with long term complications with internal hernias, with marginal ulcers, bleeding ulcers, malnutrition, malnourishment, vitamin deficiencies. I can keep on going. You get the point.

Gastric sleeve, on the other hand, it's a very fast procedure. It's a procedure that, in our practice, takes about 25 minutes to complete. It does not have all those complications I mentioned above. We don't bypass the intestine, therefore there is no rerouting of intestines or places of internal hernias happening down the road. There's nothing of that stuff. I truly believe 100% on the gastric sleeve. That is why I have written several books on the gastric sleeve and focus my practice on this procedure.

Do you perform hiatal hernia

repair without fundoplication?

A hiatal hernia, just as a quick note, it's a gap between your thorax and your abdomen. Part of your stomach is sliding into your thorax. We pull it back into place. It's left with a little gap. We close it up and we don't do fundoplication because actually part of the stomach is going to be removed as part of the gastric sleeve. We do calibrate that hiatus, that hole, that gap, which is a natural gap, calibrate it to a nice opening for food and the esophagus to come down. The rest of the stomach, as part of the gastric sleeve, is removed. There is no chance to perform a fundoplication.

Now, back in the 90s, 2000s, 2010s, the procedure of a Nissen fundoplication was indicated for patients with GERD, gastroesophageal reflux disease. Those patients went into a procedure called fundoplication. We went in laparoscopically, fixed the hiatal hernia and plicate the stomach, wrap the stomach around itself to prevent the heartburn, the reflux. In this case it's totally different. We are going into an abdomen to perform a gastric sleeve, but at the same time we find a hiatal hernia. We fix it up for the patient and we perform the gastric sleeve surgery.

Chapter 72

Staple Lines, Reflux & Probiotics

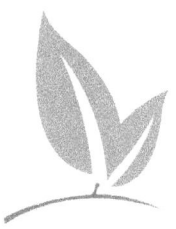

"The reason we give you these guidelines, is not to give you a hard time, it's because there's a reason for everything."

To watch the #AskDrA Show episode that this chapter is based on, follow along at: www.bit.ly/AskDrA72

Is it possible to eat something early on that could cause your staple line to rupture?

So can you eat something that may damage your staple line? If you eat something, it's not the staple line, it's not the staples, it's the timing. Please understand it's the timing. There are some guidelines you need to follow. You need to follow your doctor's guidelines. If he or she says "Clear liquids." Do clear liquids. If he or she says, "Now it's time for full liquids." It's time for full liquids. "Now it's time for soft food." Now it's time for regular food. "Now it's time for regular food." Blah blah blah, so on, so forth, you get the picture.

If you decide that it's okay to take a bite here or there while you're doing fluids or liquids or soft food, and you eat something that's not on your guideline, it is very important for you to understand that you're putting not just the staple line at risk, you're putting your health at risk, your life at risk and it is not worth it. That tiny bite that you might say, "Oh it's nothing. My staples are made from titanium. They'll hold." It's not the staples. It's your tissue. The staples are holding your tissue, recent sleeve, if make your stomach to work harder when it's not ready, you may get a leak.

The reason we give you these guidelines, is not to give you a hard time, it's because there's a reason for everything, because liquids will flow through the sleeve without putting too much tension on the healing process. Please follow your doctor's guidelines.

Would you recommend the gastric sleeve for someone with reflux?

Is the gastric sleeve recommended on somebody with reflux? Reflux is not an absolute contraindication to getting a gastric sleeve. If the reflux is studied, and the patient is taking some medication, it is not an absolute in having a gastric sleeve.

There are several reasons of heartburn. It may be a hiatal hernia that can be fixed. We had one recently actually. A patient came in for a gastric sleeve. She had a little bit of reflux. We went in. Fixed the big hiatal hernia. Gave her a sleeve. Beautiful surgery. A patient may have a hiatal hernia that may cause a reflux. Patients, may have a large belly, which is common, that increases the intra-abdominal pressure that causes reflux, so on, so forth. We need to figure out what is the possible cause, and see if the sleeve is feasible.

Do we need a probiotic?

The answer is no. That's simple. It's not needed. If you do, or are used to taking a probiotic, can you take it? The answer is yes, but it's not a necessary obligated thing to do.

Chapter 73

Eating and Drinking, Lowest BMI & Restrictions

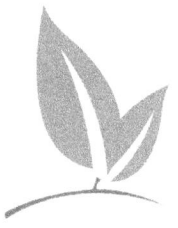

"Just remind yourself that you're not putting yourself at risk, and it's ideal to spread out the eating and drinking while you're sitting down to eat your lunch."

To watch the #AskDrA Show episode that this chapter is based on, follow along at: www.bit.ly/AskDrA73

I keep forgetting not to eat and drink at the same time. What would you recommend?

If you eat and drink after surgery, and you tolerate it, well good for you. But, if you don't tolerate it, you'll feel a very uncomfortable sensation where that liquid is trying to come down, and that food is trying to change position inside your sleeve. Feels fairly weird and uncomfortable in some patients.

What can you do? Well, practically nothing. You need to concentrate on that, but if let's say if you do forget, and you do try it out, and you feel that uncomfortable sensation, believe me, you will not forget next time. Just remind yourself that you're not putting yourself at risk, and it's ideal to spread out the eating and drinking while you're sitting down to eat your lunch. Try to stop drinking fluids, let's say 30-45 minutes before sitting down to eat, and restart your fluids 30 to 45 minutes after you finish eating.

What is the lowest BMI to be eligible for the gastric sleeve?

So the lowest BMI by criteria is normally 35, those with BMIs under 35 are evaluated on a case by case basis. Those under 35 need to exhibit other medical conditions that would show they would benefit by having weight loss surgery.

I had my VSG three days ago, and I feel like I have no restriction eating broth. Is that normal?

So you just had surgery, and are on phase 1 doing clear liquids, and you tried to do the broth, but you don't feel the restriction. Is it okay? Is the sleeve done correctly? It's normal. Keep in mind that the stomach has an entrance where food goes in, and it also has an exit where it goes to your intestine. It does not have a door on the bottom, or a barrier to stop the fluid. That's why we tell you drink clear liquids, teas, juices, broth, Gatorade, Propel Water, so on so forth. That liquid will go down through the tube, down through the sleeve without putting much restriction on it. That's what we want.

Once you finish your healing phases, and you're able to eat again, then is when you will start feeling the restriction and the capacity difference than before surgery.

Chapter 74

How Long To Heal, Can The Sleeve Be Reset & Effectiveness Long Term

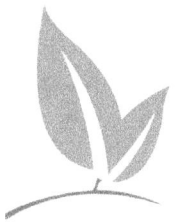

"The more effort you put in, the more magnified results you'll see."

To watch the #AskDrA Show episode that this
chapter is based on, follow along at:
www.bit.ly/AskDrA74

How long will my stomach take to heal?

For the stomach to heal correctly, it normally takes between 14 to 21 days. That is the reason we always, at least with our practice, keep you on a special diet regimen for three weeks, which is the 21 days. After 21 days, we start to eat soft food, and we progress from there. The first three weeks, it's only liquids. Anything that's solid is not permitted. That is the time where the stomach is healing side to side until it's covered with the scar tissue, and that is your own stomach. That is when it's okay to proceed and start to eat safely.

How can I reset my sleeve to lose weight again?

Well, the thing is... the sleeve is done. It's not like you need to reset it. It's not a computer you can reboot your sleeve. The sleeve is already to a certain calibration, to a certain diameter, to a certain capacity. But what you can do is put some effort on what you're filling your sleeve with. I've seen some very weird stuff online like resetting your sleeve with a five-day pouch test where people are putting in some yogurt and then some oatmeal and then just weird stuff. It really can't reset your sleeve because the sleeve is already to a certain diameter, to a certain calibration, to a certain size your surgeon left it.

What you can do is two things.

Number one - make wise decisions on what you're putting inside your sleeve. Focus on healthier stuff, fruits, vegetables, and fill your sleeve up with that stuff instead of really high carbs or high calorie concentrated food. Try to avoid all that. Healthier decisions.

Number two is increase your activity level, aka, exercise.

The more effort you put in, the more magnified results you'll see.

Don't see it as a reset button. Think about it as small changes that will give you good results down the road.

Will the sleeve still be effective after five years?

The answer is yes. The stomach will never, ever be the original size it was because it is calibrated. We cut out a good chunk of stomach, by the way, if you haven't followed me on SnapChat, that we normally fill out big stomachs, and the portion we cut out of the stomach, we fill it up with some water, so you can see how big and how much food you really need to fill up your stomach.

Down the road, the answer is yes. You will always have that tool available for you down the road. I've got patients that are 10, 11 years out, and are still doing fantastic, but it's not just the procedure. It also has to do with you, good choices, good follow-up, following the guidelines, and you'll be just fine. It's not just a tool. You have to do a lot with it.

Chapter 75

Trouble Foods, Advice Before Surgery & Why Mexico

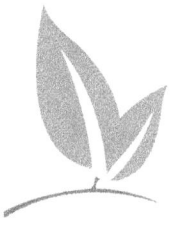

"I want to give you a much better quality healthcare, more personalized, but at an affordable cost."

To watch the #AskDrA Show episode that this chapter is based on, follow along at: www.bit.ly/AskDrA75

Is it normal that we don't tolerate some food after surgery? Like chicken?

Yeah, it's common that certain types of food, specifically chicken, really dry chicken or turkey, may give you some trouble after surgery. This is totally normal. It's expected. It's not that it's you. It's not that it's something's wrong with you. The thing is that very dry meat, like chicken or chicken breast doesn't go down as well as if you were let's say to consume chicken in the soup, or chicken that is a little bit moisty, that will go down a little bit better.

It's normal. If you change that consistency of the chicken, it will change. The thing is, remember that sleeve, it's a very narrow tube. That dry chicken stays there for a little longer time. Don't worry. It's not that something's wrong. If you're only having trouble with the chicken, don't worry, the sleeve is perfect. Try to change the consistency or the moisture of it.

Any last bits of advice before I go to surgery?

It's a no-brainer. Number one, you're going to have a procedure that's going to change your life.

Number two, it's something that's going to work so well, you're going to be losing a lot of weight, a lot of inches, a lot of sizes. You're going to be feeling so much better. It's going to increase your quality of life. It's a procedure that is known to give you good weight control down the road.

You're going to avoid, if not cure, certain conditions like high blood pressure, diabetes, cholesterol, triglycerides, sleep apnea, the snoring, knees, ankles, swollen feet. I mean, I can go on and on. It really is a no-brainer. Don't worry. Jump. Take the step. You'll be very happy with the journey.

Why are the surgeries performed in Mexico and not the US?

The reason I practice in Mexico is for you. We are able to cut down on hospital prices versus the US. I did some training in the US, and believe me, I know how prices are, just crazy. I mean, when they use a band-aid, they'll bill you for the whole box at a very expensive price.

Here in Mexico, we're able to cut down on the hospital prices. We're able to pass those savings onto you. We're able to do more surgeries. We're able to help out more people at a more affordable price.

Doesn't mean we are doing things wrong. Doesn't mean we're doing things differently, as in the States. We do sleeves exactly as if you were in Houston or Los Angeles, or New York City, or you name it. We have all the credentials, or even better credentials as requested as in the States. The reason is, my policy is I want to give you a much better quality healthcare, more personalized, but at an affordable cost. That's why, because of you.

Chapter 76

Hitting A Stall, Unflavored Protein & Preparing For Surgery

"This is a 12 to 18-month process. It's not magic. You've got to give it some time."

To watch the #AskDrA Show episode that this
chapter is based on, follow along at:
www.bit.ly/AskDrA76

Is it normal to hit a stall in weight loss when you change from liquids to solid food after surgery?

The answer is yes. The reason is you've been doing a pre-op diet, then you did a diet after surgery and you probably lost quite a bit of weight. Your body is going under an adjustment and you'll hit a stall. It's not that you just jump from clear liquids or full liquids to eating regular food, solid food, and you are noticing that you hit a stall. It's not because you've switched, it's because you've lost quite a bit on the get go and your body is adjusting. That's totally normal. Remember to have patience. This is a 12 to 18-month process. It's not magic. You've got to give it some time.

Would you suggest having clear protein or shakes post-surgery?

Flavorless protein or even the clear protein, the bullets. Do I recommend them? Can you use them?

The answer is yes. They're really good supplements, especially on the clear liquid phase, which is phase one. Those first seven days, it's a really good way to put a little bit of protein in your body. There's also the flavorless protein powder that you can mix with some broth, you can mix it up with some drinkable yogurt and it works really good as well.

Remember on phase two you can kick in with some protein shakes and other types of protein supplements.

What should I be doing now to prepare for my surgery in the spring?

Let's say, it's the beginning of the year and you're thinking of having your surgery in the spring or summer, what can you do to prepare yourself? Do not gain any more weight. In fact, you want to lose a little bit. You need to shrink your liver, and the way to do that is to lose a little bit of weight. Exercise. Watch what you eat. Cut down on the carbs, but the most important thing is, do not gain weight.

What we hear quite often, "Ah, I'm getting weight loss surgery in summer or in spring so I'll eat whatever I want. Doesn't matter. I'm going to lose weight anyway." What happens is your body weight goes up, then when you're placed on a liquid diet, your body weight comes down. That yo-yo'ing is not good for your body.

So, bottom line...do not gain weight. Try to lose the weight.

What medical tests do you need to do before surgery?

The answer is your surgeon will let you know. If you're coming to us, we do the blood work. We perform an EKG and chest-ray among other tests.

Chapter 77

Vitamins, Ketosis & Converting A Gastric Bypass To A Sleeve

After sleeve surgery intake of food is drastically reduced and it is recommended that you take a supplement."

To watch the #AskDrA Show episode that this chapter is based on, follow along at: www.bit.ly/AskDrA77

After being sleeved, if there are no malabsorption issues like bypass patients have, why is there a need to take vitamins?

The reason is because of the amount of food you consume. Before having surgery, you might have consumed, let's say on a scale of one to ten...a ten. Now after surgery you'll be eating at about a three. That means that the intake of food is drastically reduced and it is recommended that you take a supplement. In this case vitamins. There is no malabsorption, since there is nothing rerouted out of the intestines. We don't mess up with the intestines at all. We don't touch them. So, absorption of nutrients is absorbed 100%.

Why do some people get ketosis after the surgery?

Well, if your body is not taking in enough calories your body starts to focus on the fat deposits that you have in your body. Which is what we want, right? We want to lose weight from that stored fat. That stored fat gets burned and you develop these ketones. Your body totally adapts to this. You won't even notice. Your body looks for energy. Looks for that fat tissue. It burns that fat tissue. At a certain level in blood you develop ketosis. Which is what we want. We want to burn fat and lose the weight. It is normal and expected on major weight loss or weight loss surgery patients.

Can a bypass be converted to a gastric sleeve?

Can a bypass be converted to a sleeve? Can a Roux-En-Y gastric bypass be converted to a sleeve? The answer is there is no need to convert to a sleeve. It just does not make sense. In theory it can be done. In practice, it is not performed. Once you have a gastric bypass, you practically burned your bridges. You have to work with that procedure.

Now, if you have a gastric sleeve already and want to convert to something else, can it be done? Yes.
It can be converted into a duodenal switch. It can be converted to a mini gastric bypass. It can be converted to a Roux-En-Y gastric bypass. But, the other way around, it can't be done.

Chapter 78

Vegan vs Vegetarian, Part-Time Vegetarian & Drains After Surgery

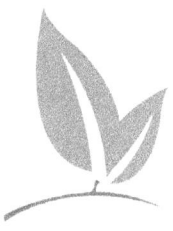

"The more vegetables you eat, and the less animal products you consume, your overall health down the road will be better."

To watch the #AskDrA Show episode that this chapter is based on, follow along at: www.bit.ly/AskDrA78

Why did you go vegan over vegetarian?

So the question is, why did I (this is more like a personal question) why did Dr. Alvarez go vegan, versus being vegetarian. Now, I did the switch from one day to the next. I'm not suggesting you do this, not everybody can. It is much simpler, if you're looking for a healthier diet, to do so in a more slowly but progressive way. You can lower your intake of animal products slowly, then you can become a vegetarian.

What's the difference between being a vegan versus a vegetarian? Vegan is completely plant- based. Being a vegetarian, you can also have eggs and some dairy products.

It's easier to become a vegetarian first, and then ultimately become a vegan, but I'm not suggesting you do this. It's simply my lifestyle. I enjoy it. I like it, but it's not something I would recommend to everybody, because it's not simple to everyone. But if you're interested, you can always contact me and I can give you some tips here and there.

How do you feel about the diets that advocate part-time vegetarian?

What do I suggest, or do I like the idea of being partially vegetarian? That means you can eat some meat or animal products, let's say, on a weekend, and then the rest of the week you could be completely vegetarian or vegan. I think it's a good way to start off, if you're interested in that lifestyle. I think the more vegetables you eat, and the less animal products you consume, your overall health down the road will be better.

Why don't you use an abdominal

drain post-surgery.

So you could have a leak, or a bleeding and if that drain is not nearby, it will not be functioning, and the patient will be presenting certain symptoms. And if the drain is clean, and nothing is coming out, you'll be thinking, "Well, everything's good, I guess. So even though I'm not feeling well, and something's going on..." But the drain is clear. So it'll be misleading.

We don't use them regularly unless there's a specific situation, maybe the patient had a previous abdominal surgery, or there was something that caught my eye and I said, "I'll just leave a drain here." But if not, we normally do not use drains. We look at different, other signs and symptoms, other things, other than just being confident on just one single drain.

That's why if you're a patient of mine, you've noticed, if you went through the Endobariatric experience with us, you noticed that we see you a lot. I have a staff of four other doctors besides myself, that we do rounds regularly. You get to see doctors around the clock, and we will check on certain things and signs and symptoms.

So that is why, in our practice, we don't use drains on every patient.

Glossary of Terms

Acid Blocker – are a class of medications that reduce or block stomach acids from forming

Acid Reflux – is a chronic condition caused by stomach acid coming up into the esophagus

Alcohol Sugar – is a carbohydrate that has fewer calories than regular sugar and less effect on blood glucose levels.

Aspirin – is a medication used to treat pain, fever, and inflammation

BMI – short for "body mass index"

Bougie – a thin flexible surgical instrument used for exploring or dilating a passage of the body

Carbs – short for "carbohydrates"

Celebrex - is a nonsteroidal anti-inflammatory drug

Creatine – a supplement used for muscle improvement.

Duodenal Switch – a weight loss surgery procedure which removes a portion of the stomach and reroutes a lengthy portion of the small intestines.

Electrolytes – a substance that produces an electrically charged solution when dissolved in water

Endoscopy - a nonsurgical procedure used to examine a person's digestive tract using an endoscope

Fluid Intake – the amount of fluid consumed daily

Glossary of Terms continued...

Gastric Bypass - refers to a surgical procedure in which the stomach is divided into a small upper pouch and a much larger lower "remnant" pouch and then the small intestine is rearranged to connect to both.

Gastric Sleeve - is a surgical weight loss procedure in which the stomach is reduced to about 25% of its original size, by surgical removal of a large portion of the stomach along the greater curvature.

GERD – is a digestive disorder that affects the lower esophageal sphincter the ring of muscle between the esophagus and stomach

Ghrelin – commonly referred to as the "hunger hormone".

Health System – an organization devoted to health care solutions.

Incision - a surgical cut made in skin or flesh.

Intestines - are a long, continuous tube running from the stomach to the anus.

IV Fluids – are liquids, medications or blood used intravenously.

Lactose Free – being free of sugars derived from milk products.

Liquid Phase – anything that has the consistency of what can easily be strained through a straw.

Malabsorption - is a state arising from abnormality in absorption of food nutrients across the GI tract.

Glossary of Terms continued...

Malnutrition - is a condition that results from eating a diet in which nutrients are not enough which then causes health problems.

Medical Tourism – is the traveling to another country to obtain medical treatment

Meloxicam – is used to treat pain or inflammation caused by rheumatoid arthritis and osteoarthritis in adults

Metabolism - is a term that is used to describe all chemical reactions involved in maintaining the living state of the cells and the organism.

NSAIDS – short for "Nonsteroidal anti-inflammatory drugs" such as aspirin, ibuprofen, naproxen

Nausea – the discomfort that you feel before vomiting

Osmolarity - the concentration of a solution expressed as the total number of solute particles per liter.

Paleo Diet – commonly referred to as the "caveman diet".

PCP - short for "primary care physician"

Restrictions – help identify a patient's limitations and capabilities.

Revisional Surgery – is a surgical procedure done to revise a past treatment.

Salt – is a combination of sodium and chlorine.

Soft Food Phase – food that has the consistency of applesauce

Glossary of Terms continued...

VSG – short for "vertical sleeve gastrectomy".

Weight Stall – is a temporary adjustment when after weight loss surgery your body stalls to lose weight.

About The Author

Dr. Guillermo Alvarez, a premier bariatric surgeon located in Piedras Negras, Coahuila, Mexico who is passionate about helping people fulfill their lifelong desire of attaining better health and a more fulfilling lifestyle. Dr. Alvarez has helped over 10,000 patients gain a new lease on life with the help of the gastric sleeve surgery.

Dr. Alvarez dedicates his practice to helping his patients achieve dramatic weight loss that leads to a healthier, longer and more prosperous life. Following weight loss surgery, many of Dr. Alvarez's patients are soon able to enjoy the benefits and joys of life that they previously could not while suffering from obesity. An improved love life, a more active lifestyle and the ability to enjoy quality time with friends and family are just some of the few positive changes that you will experience after weight loss surgery.

Endobariatric

Dr. Alvarez's bariatric surgery Mexico facility is updated frequently to stay ahead of the normal standards used in the USA. The operating room is equipped with an emergency power plant that guarantees continuous electrical supply in case of an emergency such as an uncommon blackout. The hospital has a wide variety of diagnostic equipment that is found in large hospitals in the States, such as an MRI, Helicoidal CT Scan, Doppler Sonogram, etc.

This hospital has the top intensive care unit in this region with a staff of doctors and nurses that specialize in any trauma or emergency to support our patients in any case needed. You can feel safe in knowing that the staff of this facility is more than capable in handling your needs as a patient. The hospital is considered a "Specialized" hospital to handle the most difficult individual cases that are present.

The hospital includes 35 private rooms for patients and guest. Each room has telephone, TV, cable and a place for your guests to sleep. There are 4 suites available that also have a sofa and recliner.

The nursing staff is very professional and well trained for your care as a bariatric patient. There are 3 shifts (as opposed to the states - 2 shifts). We feel that is important that our entire team is fresh and alert to keep a 24-hour monitoring protocol. This entire staff is more than capable in handling all of your post-op care.

This hospital is a wonderful place for our bariatric patients to experience a safe and calm atmosphere and an excellent outcome during your recovery period. If you are considering this surgery for yourself or a family member, feel free to contact us any time. This is an option that will ensure you the best care from an excellent team of surgeons, nurses and top-notch hospital. We will be happy to have one of our coordinators assist you with more information and pricing.

1(866)697-5338 www.Endobariatric.com

Endo-Spa

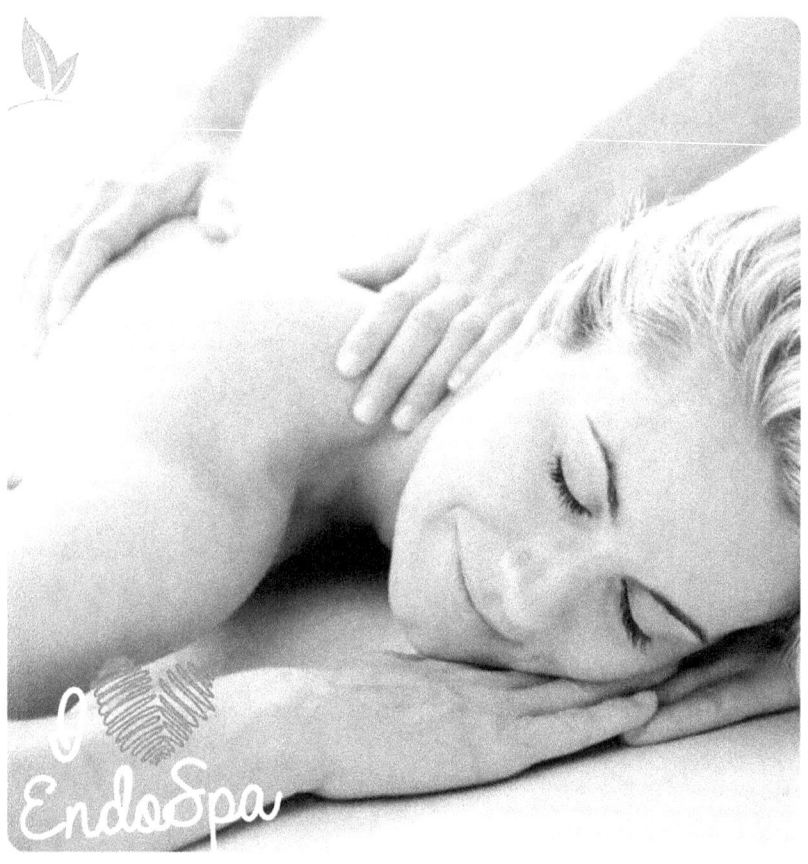

With relaxing surroundings, innovative treatments and a talented staff, EndoSpa nurtures your body, invigorates your senses and relaxes your mind. EndoSpa offers a wide array of spa treatments for men and women.

Massage – Facials – Laser Treatment Hair Removal –

Acoustic Wave Therapy

www.EndoSpa.mx

Endo-Store

- Shirts
- Hats
- Bags
- Bottles
- Pillows
- Books

And more!

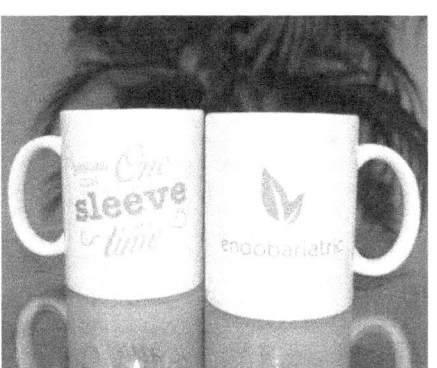

www.EndoStoreOnline.com

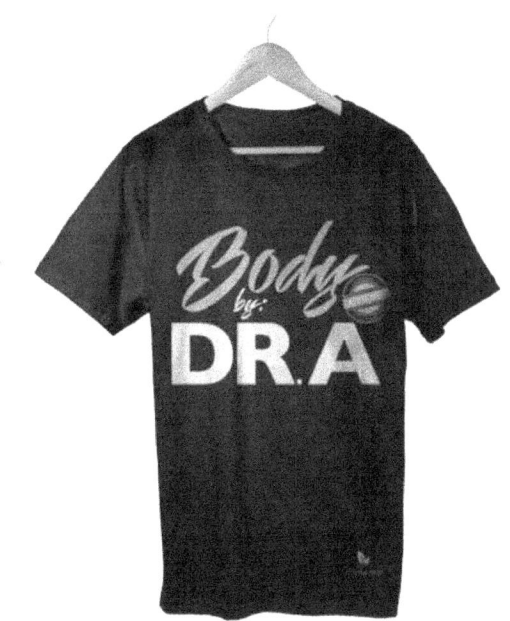

The Book That Started The Series

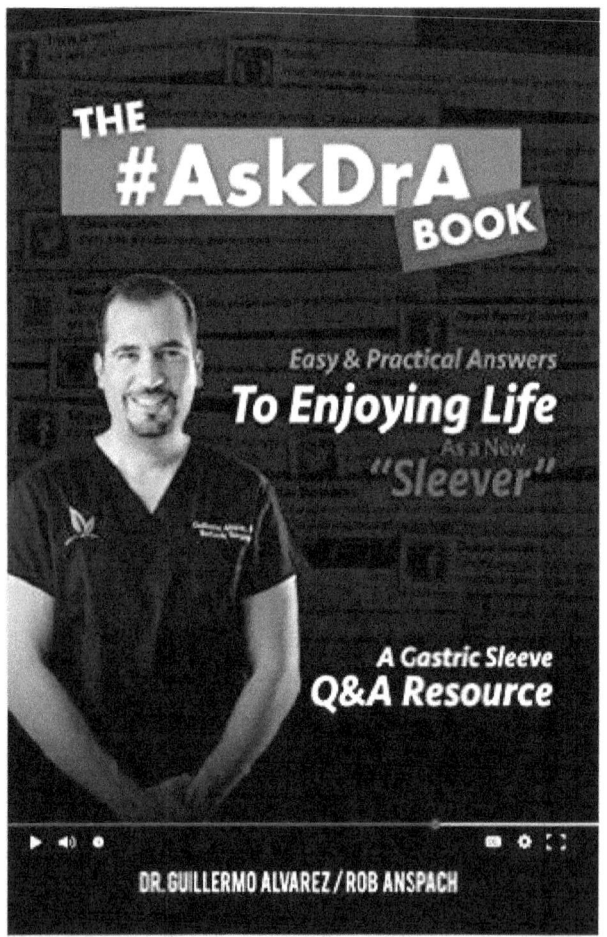

Available on Amazon & EndoStoreOnline.com

Other Books By
Dr. Guillermo Alvarez

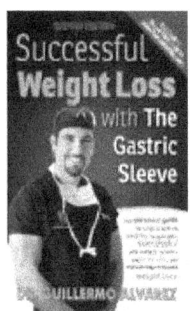 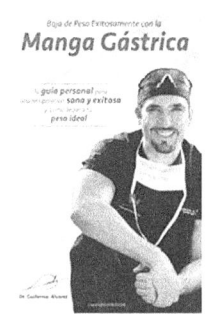 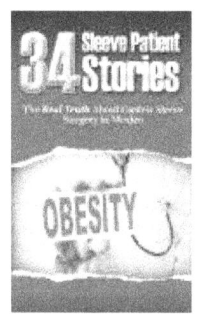

Available on Amazon

Be A Fan!

Follow Dr. Alvarez on these Social Networks

Facebook - www.facebook.com/endobariatric

Google+ - https://plus.google.com/+Endobariatric

Twitter - www.twitter.com/endobariatric

Pinterest - www.pinterest.com/endobariatric

Instagram - www.instagram.com/endobariatric

LinkedIn - www.linkedin.com/in/endobariatric

YouTube - www.youtube.com/endobariatric

Snapchat - www.snapchat.com/add/gmoalvarez

If you have a question and would like to get it answered...post it to Facebook, Twitter, Instagram or YouTube with the hashtag #AskDrA

Or send your question via Snapchat.

We might even answer it on our weekly show or in the next book.

Share This Book!

I mean it!

Tell your friends all about this book.

Share where you bought it.

Share it at lunch! Share it at the gym! Share it on the beach!

Share it on social media.

Share it using this hashtag...

#TheAskDrABook3

www.ingramcontent.com/pod-product-compliance
Lightning Source LLC
Chambersburg PA
CBHW052325220526
45472CB00001B/270